Published By Adam Gilbin

@ Tony Dodd

Successful Life: Powerful Methods to Create

Motivation, Energy, Vitality and Soulfulness How

to Lead a Successful Life

All Right RESERVED

ISBN 978-87-94477-60-4

TABLE OF CONTENTS

chapter 1 1

Self-Discovery 1

Chapter 2 12

Power Of Experiential Learning 12

To Get A Phd In Results, Pursue Realisation Over
Understanding. 12

Chapter 3 27

Personal Finances And Banking 27

Chapter 4 31

The Mindset's Power To Create Wealth 31

Chapter 5 38

Your Professional Decline Is Coming Sooner Than You
Think 38

Chapter 6 45

How A Problem Solver Thinks 45

Chapter 7 72

The Science Of Habits- Unraveling The Marvels Of Your
Brain's Habitual Symphony 72

Chapter 8	80
Forging Resilience And Growth	80
Chapter 9	90
Finding Personal Success And Fulfilment	90
Chapter 10	98
Emotional Intelligence	98
Chapter 11	116
Clearly Defined Financial Objectives	116
Chapter 12	123
Kick Your Success Addiction	123
Chapter 13	131
The Discovery Process Of Problem Solving	131

Chapter 1

Self-Discovery

Embrace Your Uniqueness

Imagine a world where everyone looked, thought, and acted the same—bland, monotonous, and devoid of excitement. Fortunately, that's not the world we live in. You are a masterpiece, a combination of experiences, interests, and talents that no one else possesses. Embrace your uniqueness like a badge of honor. It's what makes you, well, you.

To truly know yourself, take a journey inward. Reflect on your passions, your dreams, and the things that make your heart race with excitement. What are your strengths? What are your weaknesses? Embracing your individuality lays the foundation for a fulfilling and authentic life.

Practical Tip: Start a Journal

Create a safe space for self-reflection. Start a journal where you can jot down your thoughts, dreams, and experiences. It's not just a record; it's a mirror reflecting the essence of who you are.

Set Boundaries

In the grand ballet of life, it's easy to get swept away by the demands and expectations of others. While being considerate of those around you is important, setting healthy boundaries is equally crucial. Understand what you value, what you stand for, and what you won't compromise. Learning to say "no" when needed is a powerful skill that protects your time, energy, and well-being.

Try Something New

Step out of your comfort zone. Whether it's a new hobby, a different route to school, or trying a new cuisine, embracing change begins with small, intentional steps outside the familiar.

Be Kind to Yourself

The journey of self-discovery is not always a smooth ride. There will be bumps, detours, and unexpected twists. In these moments, be kind to yourself. Understand that mistakes are stepping stones, not stumbling blocks. Treat yourself with the same compassion and understanding you offer to your closest friends.

The Power of a Polite

Practice saying "no" assertively but politely. It's a skill that takes time to develop, but once mastered, it becomes a shield against unnecessary stress and obligations.

Embrace Change

Life is a series of constant transformations. Embracing change is not just about adapting; it's about evolving. Each experience, whether positive or challenging, shapes you into a more resilient and adaptable individual. Change is the sculptor; you are the masterpiece in the making.

Positive Affirmations

Start and end your day with positive affirmations. Remind yourself of your strengths, acknowledge your efforts, and express gratitude for the unique qualities that make you who you are.

Weekly Check-ins

Set aside a specific time each week for self-reflection. It could be a quiet Sunday evening or a Wednesday morning ritual. Use this time to assess your progress, celebrate achievements, and recalibrate your course if needed.

Cultivate Self-Reflection

Self-discovery is an ongoing process. Take time regularly to reflect on your experiences, your growth, and your goals. What have you learned? How have you changed? What do you aspire to become? Self-reflection is the compass that keeps you moving in the right direction.

Embracing Individuality

The journey to self-discovery is not a solo expedition—it's a collaborative venture between who you are and who you want to become. Embracing your individuality is not just about understanding yourself; it's about celebrating the diversity of those around you.

Celebrate Differences

The world is a rich tapestry woven with threads of diverse cultures, perspectives, and backgrounds. Celebrate the differences that make each person unique. Learn from others, listen to their stories, and appreciate the beauty of a world painted in a myriad of colors.

Cultural Exchange

Explore cultural events, try different cuisines, and engage in conversations with people from diverse backgrounds. This not only broadens your horizons but also fosters a deep appreciation for the richness of human diversity.

Respect Others' Opinions

Just as you have your own thoughts and beliefs, so do others. Respecting diverse opinions is a cornerstone of healthy relationships and societal harmony. It's okay to disagree, but do so respectfully, recognizing that differing perspectives contribute to a vibrant and dynamic world.

Practical Tip: Empathetic Listening

Practice empathetic listening when engaging in discussions. Seek to understand before being understood. It not only fosters respect but also opens the door to meaningful conversations.

Nurture Empathy

Empathy is the ability to understand and share the feelings of another. It's a superpower that connects hearts and builds bridges. Cultivate empathy by putting yourself in others' shoes, by actively listening, and by responding with kindness and understanding.

Practical Tip: Random Acts of Kindness

Make kindness a daily habit. Whether it's holding the door open for someone, offering a genuine compliment, or simply being present for a friend in need, small acts of kindness amplify the bonds that connect us all.

Be a Lifelong Learner

The beauty of individuality lies in its ever-evolving nature. As you discover more about yourself, remember that growth is a continuous process. Be a lifelong learner, open to new ideas, experiences, and perspectives. The more you learn, the more you enrich your own narrative.

Explore New Hobbies

Dabble in hobbies you've never tried before. Whether it's painting, coding, or playing a musical instrument, exploring new interests opens up avenues for self-discovery and personal growth.

Express Yourself

Your individuality is like a kaleidoscope of colors waiting to be seen. Express yourself authentically—through art, music, writing, or any medium that resonates with you. Your unique voice adds to the symphony of human expression.

Creative Outlets

Discover your creative outlets and make them a regular part of your routine. Whether it's journaling, creating digital art, or playing an instrument, find ways to express your thoughts, emotions, and ideas.

Closing this chapter of self-discovery, remember that the journey is ongoing. You are an evolving masterpiece, and each day is a stroke on the canvas of your life. As you continue exploring the intricacies of who you are, cherish the adventure, embrace the unknown, and celebrate the vibrant tapestry of your individuality.

Embrace Collaboration

Life is a team sport. Whether you're working on a school project, participating in sports, or engaging in group activities, collaboration is a skill that propels you forward. Recognize the strengths of others, contribute your unique talents, and watch the magic unfold when diverse minds come together.

Team Building Activities

Participate in team-building exercises or group projects. These experiences not only enhance your collaboration skills but also provide opportunities to learn from others and discover new aspects of yourself.

Chapter 2

Power of Experiential Learning

To get a PhD in Results, pursue realisation over understanding.

I am a great proponent of Experiential Learning.

Let's take an example. If I asked you to recite a poem you learned in your KG class, you could do it without any problem. All of us can do it. However, if I ask you to recite a poem from your 8th standard, I bet most of us will not be able to recall it. The difference in the recall is only in the way of teaching. In KG, when the teacher taught you 'I am a little teapot', she made you act like a teapot, with a giant rendering of a teapot attached to you, with a handle and a spout.

A good teacher may even give you a taste of a cup of tea. This teaching technique involves all five senses. The more senses are involved, the better the recall, simply because all five senses give you an experience, and that experience is unique to you. The learning from such an experience goes into what is called cellular memory. Hence the recall is for life. On the other hand, as we start growing, the studying pattern is more about memorising, which resides in our brain memory. Hence the recall is terrible. I am not suggesting that understanding is not essential. The linear way of learning is first to understand and then apply. This book presents Experiential Learning, where you first apply and then make learnings out of that.

Let me give you the Adult Learning process **used in competency development. The process has four stages:**

- Conscious Competence
- Unconscious Competence
- Unconscious Incompetence
- Conscious Incompetence

Let's take the competency of riding a bicycle. Those who don't know about cycling can relate it to swimming, car driving, or even learning to walk. When you are reading this, go through your own relevant experience.

At one point, you had no idea what a cycle was; at that point, you were unconscious of your incompetence in how to cycle. Since you were unaware of this incompetency, —you were leading a happy life. Remember, no one likes the word incompetent.

One fine day, you went to your school and saw your friend arriving on a cycle. At that moment, you became conscious of your incompetence. This stage is important because the moment you become conscious of your incompetence, it creates a drive in you. **The stronger the drive, the faster the learning.**

Feeling incompetent, you went home and started crying and howling for a cycle. You wanted a cycle. So you either hired or bought one. Let's assume that you purchased one. When you unboxed it, it came with an A4 sheet of paper titled "This is How You Ride a Cycle". This page consists of 10 simple steps on how to cycle. Now, if I said I give you 24 hours to memorise these ten steps thoroughly, after 24 hours, I will test you. Would you score 10/10? I bet you would. With ten simple steps to memorise in 24 hours, anyone can achieve a ten on 10. The golden question, however, is whether you will be able to cycle. The answer is a big NO.

So what you did was you sat on the cycle with the help of either your dad or mom and started pedalling. Initially, you struggled; however, your drive did not allow you to give up. Maybe you fell at times and had bruises, cuts, and some blood here and there—all of this did not matter. You kept on going. Suddenly, one day, there was a time when you did not know that your dad or mom had stopped holding behind you; unaware of it, you went on pedalling like crazy, realising in a flash of a second that you were on your own, no dad, no mom, no one holding you. Remember that exhilarating, exciting moment? There was an **internal shift** in you when you realised you now know how to cycle.

What you learned about how to cycle was one single word: **Balance**. You learned how to balance the cycle. Here is a quick question for all of you: Can you teach this balance to anyone? The answer is a big NO because it is an experience. It is impossible to teach this to just anyone. Experience is an individual phenomenon and hence cannot be taught. It is a reality that an individual has to learn it all by himself. This learning, this realisation, comes from within. You realised how to balance the cycle, not just understand.

I bet many of you last sat on a cycle long ago. If I give you a cycle right now, can you ride it? You may struggle for a few seconds, but that's fine. But you will be able to cycle. I can see the smiles on your faces. The answer is YES. **What you**

learned in a fraction of a second remains with you for life. This is the importance of Experiential Learning. That is why you must learn to apply all the life learnings, whether through this book or from anywhere.

Note, however, that the competency is still at the Conscious stage. Remember how you were at that stage: your body was tight, tense, purely focused on cycling, not looking here or there. The competency still has to go unconscious. That's where stage 4 comes into play.

This is an important stage for any adult to make the competence unconscious. **Repetition is the only answer to mastery in this competency**. You were so excited that you cycled daily, and the magic happened in a couple of days or months. At some stage in your practice, you no longer need to think about how to cycle. If anyone woke you up in the middle of the night or stuffed in a few pegs of alcohol, you could still cycle. Thinking is no longer needed. The competency has gone into your unconscious. You have mastered the art of cycling.

It is the same with all life learning. Once you receive any life learning from any place, your job is to take **massive action** on it; that is, if you wish to retain the knowledge for life. Implementing life learning gives you only two results: a pass or a fail. Both are learning lessons in the process that I have designed, so there is a double benefit. Action is imperative to bring about any change, hence the insistence on implementation. You write a Personal Action plan in any area where you wish for breakthrough or better results. Visit my YouTube channel and watch the Action Plan and Implementation Playlist, with which you will completely understand how to utilise your life learnings.

Here is my story of how I learned to apply the same.

The story of how I stopped smoking.

The whole world understands that smoking is injurious to health. But how many people stop smoking? Even the gory pictures on the packet do not deter some of them. I have been a smoker, and there was a time in my life when I smoked 30 cigarettes a day. A friend of mine and I always had conversations about quitting. Both of us had tried all sorts of tricks to quit, such as smoking half a cigarette, buying only one cigarette at a time, and using various filters and nicotine patches, with no success rate. I was once successful with nine months of no smoking. Then, a few of my friends and their families decided to go to Goa for a vacation. One of these friends was a smoker. I remember that day; we were all sitting and enjoying a few drinks when he went out for a smoke. I tried to avoid it all for some time but was eventually left alone in the room. So I joined them. He casually said, "Come on, Raju, have a drag." During vacation, our guards are usually down, as mine was. I said to myself, it's okay if I take just one drag. In that weak moment, I took that one drag. In the next two days, I was back to my smoking. The point is that I was committed to quitting smoking, which helped me try different ways, though the success rate was pathetic. But I did not give up.

My friend & I were multi-level marketing distributors to a health and wellness company named Herbalife and were selected for leadership training in Bangalore. We were in a vast hall with some 300-odd distributors. At the time, I was putting a lot of effort into the business; however, the returns were not up to expectations, and frustration was setting in. One of the sessions was conducted by a Japanese American who was speaking, and as he spoke, I connected to it; it was as if he were talking about my life.

He said you guys are in this room, meaning you have a dream. Write your dream down on the notepad. I did. With this, he started sharing his life in the organisation and how he was frustrated; despite the efforts that he was putting in, he was not getting the desired results. He said once, after a long flight, he reached the hotel late at night, exhausted. He said I was cursing my local downline as they had arranged for an early morning meeting. I was in no mood to attend the meeting, but my dream did not allow me to sleep, and I got up early. Sitting with a cup of coffee, I saw myself in the huge full-length mirror. One thought crossed my mind; he said, if I hired the person in the mirror, with the exact amount that I was dreaming about, write down what I would expect that person to do. He said that in the next ten minutes, I had two A4 pages full of my expectations written down. He said the bigger shock was that I was not doing even one of them.

Mentally, I did the same exercise, and when I found myself in the same situation, I asked myself whether I was serious about the business. The answer within, I was. At this point in the workshop, my internal voice said, "Raju, here you are talking about health and wellness to people, and you smoke on the sly; who will listen to you, and why should anyone listen to you?" Something in me shifted internally at that moment, and from then on, I dropped smoking. I have lost count of how many years ago this was. However, friends, let me tell you, from that moment till this moment, I have not thought about smoking, nor even any desire to. I have not had any withdrawal symptoms since then, either. It seems magical now. Like everyone, I <u>understood</u> that smoking is injurious to health, yet I smoked. It was only when I <u>realised</u> that smoking is injurious to health that it caused such a massive transformation.

Life Learning
These are tried and time-tested concepts and strategies which have worked for millions of people who have learned to apply them, not just understand them. Understanding is easy, but cannot make a difference in your life. If you want the best results, learn to apply whatever appeals to you from the book. It is in the application that you will find your results and answers. All my life learning is highlighted in italics in this book for your ease.

I heard somewhere that information that is not applied is garbage. It's so true. If you want to enhance your VIP (what VIP means is detailed further in Chapter 6), position yourself in life, or stand out, you must apply everything you have learned. **Results are the only way to influence others**, whether children, peers, bosses, or anyone else. You have heard of PhD finance, PhD marketing, and more. But have you heard of a PhD in Results? Through my program, I teach people to be a master in producing results. I tell people I have a PhD in producing results, and so can you.

Implementation of knowledge is the only way to achieve your PhD in Results.

Pause from time to time, reflect on your life and connect the life learning shared in the book with your own experiences. Identify places in life where you can apply this learning. Apply, and learn from your application.

Exercise

The way to apply the learning from this chapter is to write a Personal Action Plan in the areas that you need to work on to get the required results and achieve balance in your life.

This is a process. For details of this process, please visit my YouTube channel. Go to the Playlist section and watch the Action Plan and Implementation Playlist.

Chapter 3

**Personal Finances
and Banking**

If you have followed the guidelines outlined in this book, congratulations on successfully obtaining a job! Whether you're just starting your journey into the workforce or already have employment, this chapter on personal finances and banking is a must-read. It covers essential aspects of managing your money, understanding financial systems, and making informed financial decisions.

Now that you have a job, it's crucial to understand the significance of personal finances. This chapter will provide you with the necessary knowledge and tools to take control of your financial well-being. It starts by emphasizing the importance of budgeting, which involves tracking your income and expenses to ensure that you live within your means. Budgeting allows you to prioritize your spending, save for the future, and avoid unnecessary debt.

In addition to budgeting, this chapter delves into the world of banking. It introduces you to different banking services and products, such as checking accounts, savings accounts, and debit cards. You will learn how to open a bank account, manage your account effectively, and utilize banking services to simplify your financial transactions.

Moreover, the next chapter sheds light on the concept of credit and its role in your financial life. Understanding credit is crucial because it affects your ability to borrow money, obtain favorable interest rates, and make significant purchases like a car or a house. Again, the next chapter will learn more about credit scores, credit reports, and how to establish and maintain good credit.

Furthermore, this chapter explores the importance of saving and investing. It discusses various saving strategies, such as setting financial goals, building an emergency fund, and planning for retirement. You will also gain insights into different investment options, such as stocks, bonds, and mutual funds, and how they can help grow your wealth over time.

Throughout this chapter, you will find practical tips, real-life examples, and advice on making wise financial decisions. By applying the knowledge and strategies presented, you will be better equipped to manage your personal finances, build financial security, and work towards your long-term financial goals.

Remember, personal finances are an integral part of adult life. Developing good financial habits early on will set you on the path to financial freedom and independence. So, whether you're just starting your career or looking to enhance your financial knowledge, this chapter will provide you with the essential information needed to make informed financial choices and pave the way for a secure financial future.

Chapter 4

The Mindset's Power to Create Wealth

The Basics of Mentality

Fundamentally, a person's mindset is their combination of attitudes and ideas that serve as a lens through which they view and understand the world. The influence of thought is evident in how people handle money, success, and abundance when it comes to creating riches. A person's financial destiny is largely determined by whether they approach financial endeavours with an abundance or scarcity mindset.

Creating the Financial Story

Take Felix as an example, whose life turns into a microcosm that highlights the importance of mentality. Felix encountered financial difficulties at a young age. Despite their resilience, his family struggled with money. Felix, on the other hand, had a different outlook: he saw obstacles as chances, failures as learning experiences, and scarcity as a blank canvas for plenty. Although the difficulties remained, this viewpoint reframed them so that they became opportunities for development rather than impassable barriers.

The Law of Attraction and Mentality

The deep relationship between attitude and the Law of Attraction is inevitably explored in an examination of mindset in wealth development. The belief that positive thinking brings financial success is based on the metaphysical principle of like attracts like in the context of finances. The chapter analyses how the energy we radiate from our ideas and convictions affects the financial possibilities and results that come our way.

Felix's Experience with Attraction Law

Felix's life turns into an example of the Law of Attraction in action. Through constant mental alignment with profitable outcomes, he drew chances that drove him to success. The chapter describes several events in Felix's life where his thinking attracted wealth, demonstrating the concrete effects of directing one's thoughts towards the desired financial outcome.

Getting Rid of Limiting Thoughts

In terms of creating money, mindset has two sides: beliefs that are empowering on the one hand and ideas that are restricting on the other. This chapter's portion examines the harmful effects of limiting beliefs, or deeply held ideas that limit one's potential financially. These beliefs, which can have their origins in early life, social indoctrination, or personal setbacks, function as imperceptible barriers that prevent people from realising their full potential financially.

Techniques for Dispelling Limiting Thoughts

Using psychological concepts and real-world examples, the chapter presents a toolkit for breaking down limiting beliefs. Through exercises in immersive visualisation and cognitive reframing, readers are guided through practical tactics to identify and get beyond mental obstacles that might be impeding their financial growth.

The Wealth Mindset's Neuroscience

In order to fully understand the role that attitude plays in creating wealth, neuroscience is being investigated. The brain, an amazing organ with the ability to rewire itself, is a major factor in determining one's financial mindset. This chapter explains how to use neuroplasticity, or the brain's capacity to create new neural connections, to develop a wealth-creating attitude.

Felix's Successfully Rewired Brain

Felix's journey, supported by scientific findings, shows how his brain pathways were rewired through intentional practises and continuous mindset interventions. The science underlying this change is uncovered in this chapter, which explores neurotransmitters, neural networks, and the influence of habits on the development of a wealth-oriented attitude.

Developing a Growth Mentality to Attract Wealth

Near the end of the chapter, the focus shifts to the idea of a growth mindset, which is a critical distinction between people who accumulate long-term wealth and those who experience financial stagnation. A growth mindset, which has its roots in the groundbreaking research of psychologist Carol Dweck, is defined by the conviction that learning and progress are possible.

Realistic Methods for Developing a Growth Mentality

Instead of being left with a theoretical understanding, readers receive practical advice on how to encourage a growth mentality. A combination of case studies, psychological concepts, and hands-on activities help people change from a fixed mindset to one that welcomes obstacles, perseveres through failures, and views hard work as the route to achievement and prosperity.

The first chapter goes beyond what is typically considered to be the limits of financial writing. It challenges readers to not just recognise but also actively participate in the significant impact that mentality has on their financial path. Felix's story, scientific investigation, and useful tactics provide a strong basis for the upcoming transformative journey, which is to acquire the attitude necessary for long-term financial success.

Chapter 5

Your Professional Decline is Coming Sooner Than You Think

Exploring the natural evolution of professional life

The natural evolution of professional life is a multifaceted journey, characterized by its inherent dynamism and transformative phases. Rather than a linear progression, it resembles a continuous cycle of growth, adaptation, and change.

At its core, this evolution acknowledges that careers unfold in stages, marked by peaks of achievement, plateaus of stability, and transitions leading to new opportunities. Embracing this cyclical nature allows individuals to appreciate the diverse experiences that contribute to the overall tapestry of their professional narrative.

Adaptability is a key theme in this evolution. Professionals are encouraged to cultivate a mindset that welcomes change, recognizing it not as a disruptor but as an essential catalyst for personal and career development. This adaptability empowers individuals to navigate uncertainties, seize new opportunities, and remain resilient in the face of challenges.

Continuous learning becomes a cornerstone of this evolution. Professionals are urged to engage in ongoing skill development, staying attuned to industry trends and emerging technologies. The commitment to learning fosters agility, ensuring that individuals remain relevant and adept in an ever-evolving professional landscape.

Exploration and openness to new opportunities are integral aspects of natural evolution.

Embracing change involves seeking fresh challenges, whether within the current role or by venturing into new professional domains. This spirit of exploration contributes to a sense of fulfillment and prevents stagnation.

Introspection plays a pivotal role in understanding the natural evolution of professional life. Regular reflection on personal goals, values, and aspirations helps individuals align their career paths with their broader life objectives. This self-awareness becomes a guiding force, steering professionals toward decisions that resonate with their authentic selves.

Ultimately, the natural evolution of professional life invites individuals to celebrate change as a positive force. By recognizing the cyclical nature of their careers, professionals can approach transitions with resilience, wisdom, and a clear sense of purpose. This journey is not about reaching a static destination but embracing the ongoing narrative of growth, adaptation, and fulfillment in the ever-changing landscape of the professional world.

Discussing the importance of recognizing and adapting to changing circumstances

Recognizing and adapting to changing circumstances is a crucial skill that underpins personal and professional success. In the dynamic landscape of life, unforeseen changes are inevitable, making the ability to acknowledge and respond to these shifts a valuable asset.

First and foremost, recognition is the foundation of effective adaptation. Acknowledging changing circumstances allows individuals to confront reality, fostering a clear understanding of the challenges or opportunities at hand. This awareness enables informed decision-making, preventing denial or resistance that may impede progress.

Adaptation is about flexibility and resilience in the face of change. Those who can adjust their strategies, perspectives, and actions in response to evolving circumstances are better positioned to navigate uncertainties successfully. This agility is especially relevant in the professional realm, where industries, technologies, and market demands are in a constant state of flux.

Moreover, adapting to change fosters innovation. It encourages individuals to explore new ideas, embrace novel approaches, and leverage emerging opportunities. This proactive mindset is a driving force behind personal and organizational growth, ensuring a capacity to thrive in dynamic environments.

In relationships, both personal and professional, the ability to adapt to changing circumstances enhances collaboration and communication. It fosters understanding and empathy, as individuals recognize the evolving needs and perspectives of others. This adaptability contributes to building resilient, interconnected communities.

From a personal development standpoint, adapting to change promotes continuous learning. Embracing new circumstances often requires acquiring new skills, broadening knowledge, and expanding one's comfort zone. This commitment to ongoing growth is integral to staying relevant and competitive in today's fast-paced world.

Recognizing and adapting to changing circumstances is not merely a skill but a mindset crucial for navigating the complexities of life. It empowers individuals to face challenges with resilience, seize opportunities with innovation, and foster meaningful connections through understanding. As an ongoing process, this recognition and adaptation lay the foundation for a dynamic and fulfilling journey through life's ever-evolving landscape.

Chapter 6

How A Problem Solver Thinks

Problem solving isn't just simply a task, rather it is a way of thinking. The Art of Problem Solving is more about a state of mind than doing any one thing. So how do problem solvers approach life? Well, they approach everything with the concept of discovery in their head. Discovery is the act of being able to sift through information and finding out the things that are relevant to the task at hand. For example, if you were trying to figure out how to fix a flat tire, what would the process of discovery look for?

The first step you're going to take in learning a solution is actually automatic. You're going to fall back on past experiences. If you've fixed flat tires before, your mind is going to quickly take you back to the time where you fixed the tire. It will inform you of all the steps involved. If you had studied on the process of how to fix a flat tire, you would recall that information.

What happens, however, when that automatic search that runs through your mind comes up empty? What do you do when you suddenly realize that you don't have an answer to your question? There are many different responses. Some people will call a knowledgeable friend for assistance while others might consult the internet. Some might just freeze up entirely, unable to figure out the next step in their problem solving path.

The process of beginning to look at solutions is known as the discovery process. There are many different ways to go about discovery, but oftentimes we become very limited in our ability to look for those solutions. What makes it so hard for us to think past these obstacles? Well, oftentimes it's because these obstacles give the appearance that they are somewhat insolvable. The reality isn't that the problem is insurmountable. The reality is that we ourselves can put great limitations on our own abilities.

The mindset of a problem solver, however, isn't one that is concerned with the inability to deal with something. Rather the mindset of the problem solver is much more interested in trying their best to solve the problem at hand. They do this by sifting through all available methods of learning and determining which is the best. In other words, they use the process of discovery until they are able to come to an adequate solution that will ultimately assist them in their goals.

So how do we frame our minds to think in terms of a problem solver? Well, since it's a state of mind, that means if you begin to develop specific habits and patterns of thought. If you constantly work to keep the frame of mind, eventually you will start becoming a problem solver of your own. Let's take a look at some of the mindsets that are behind the thought process of the problem solver.

Confidence in Learning

A problem solver's mind is geared in such a way that they know they have the capacity to learn the answer, even if they don't have the answer readily available. By developing the skill set to learn how to solve a problem, they are capable of figuring out exactly what is necessary to fix the situation. Let's look at a very common form of problem solving: fixing a computer.

When it comes to fixing a computer, most people feel very helpless. Oftentimes they will consult with problem solvers to fix said machine. If their email isn't working or if something goes wrong with the software, a person can be quick to call a friend who is "good with computers." This person who is supposedly good with computers usually has access to one secret that the ordinary personal doesn't know. That secret? Google. Believe it or not, but most computer gurus know that there are potentially thousands of problems that can occur when it comes to computers. There are so many issues at hand that knowing the exact answer to a problem isn't nearly as valuable as knowing how to find the answer.

A computer specialist's job is more about finding the correct solution than knowing it off of the top of his head. When he goes to his friend's house to fix the computer, he most likely is going to either operate purely off of experience if he's seen the issue a few times before or just run a quick search about what the problem is. His ability to use the search function and learn how to solve the problem makes him the most capable individual in that house when it comes to problem solving.

If the distressed computer user would spend time learning the process of going to search for solutions and how to consistently sift through data until a solution was reached, they'd be quite capable of being just as skilled with computers as the specialist.

A problem solver's job isn't to know everything, because frankly that is impossible. Rather the problem solver works to cultivate a mindset of readiness to learn. They focus on gaining the ability to learn instead of trying to just memorize everything necessary to solve a problem. This might seem a little confusing, the idea of learning how to learn. But consider this: college students who take a class on how to learn will outperform college students who don't take the class over the course of a year.

We often take the concept of learning for granted. It can be incredibly easy to just assume that you know how to learn well and then move onto other, more pressing matters. The fact might be that if you are struggling with the Art of Problem Solving, this could be an education issue. By spending some time learning how to learn well, you will be setting yourself up for success.

A problem solver has confidence in the ability to learn the answer. This essentially takes away one of the most intimidating things a problem often provides: the unknown. If you are confident that you can spend time learning the answer to problems, instead of being confident in your ability to know the problems ahead of time, you don't have to worry about the fear of the unknown. You can just focus on learning the answers to the questions that you have.

Here are some tips for adapting the mindset of Confidence in Learning:

- Don't let your lack of education on a subject daunt you. You can spend adequate time learning about the subject through books, online videos, college level courses if you're really committed or just asking a friend who knows about it.

- Humility is the key when it comes to adapting a learning mindset. It takes a certain amount of guts to be able to say, "I don't know the answer." So, in order to truly spend time Never say, I don't know. Rather try to find the answer somehow.
- In today's information driven society, you are far more capable of learning the intimate workings of something just by looking it up online.
- learning how to solve your problems, you're going to need the humility to learn from other sources about the situation.

Humility

While it is very easy to ask others for input into our ideas and concepts, it can actually be a little harder to just agree and take their advice at face value. Oftentimes when it comes to our own selves, we have to deal with our ego and pride. We are constantly trying to prove that we are capable on our own. Yet a problem solver doesn't give into pride. They are willing to lower themselves through the act of humility and truly consider what others have to tell them.

Just as we talked about learning the ability to gain information on the subject at hand, we would like for you to know that there is a great number of people in this world who can help you in solving your problems. There is a myth that in order to be successful in life we must make it through all of our problems and obstacles alone. That accepting help somehow makes us weaker. In truth, looking to others in our times of need makes us much stronger because we have the assistance of another person to help carry the workload.

It takes humility to reach out to others and ask them for their advice. Saying "I can't figure this out alone" can feel somewhat scary, especially if we have to admit it to our superiors in the workplace. But a problem solver is more interested in solving the issue at hand than keeping his own pride. Think about it, when it comes to solving problems, what is the ultimate goal? Is the goal to feel really good about ourselves and think about how great we are? Or is the goal to actually solve the problem? Someone who refuses to reach out for assistance from others is just trying to feed their own egos. A real problem solver focuses on what needs to be solved and calls out for help quickly and eagerly.

Resilience

Resilience is the fine art of being able to spring back from a difficulty. The concept of a resilient person would be like the boxer who, after being walloped hard in the face, is able to sufficiently recover from the blow and begin fighting back against his opponent.

A problem solver is resilient in the face of adversity. There are times when a problem solver can become overwhelmed or frustrated. There will be discouragement in the life of a problem solver and they can certainly be tempted to give up. They might even stop trying for a little bit, but in the end they bounce back. They are resilient.

Likewise, if we want to develop the mindset of being a problem solver, it means that we must develop a firm and strong form of resilience. We need an inner strength that allows us to come back from frustrations and poor situations with strength and determination. So how do we develop a resilient mind? Well, it requires discipline and dedication but it also requires a sense of optimism. If you don't have the ability to see that things will get better, how can you ever expect to bounce back?

Problem solving isn't about simply just fixing something. Remember, it is about developing a powerful mindset that allows you to systematically approach any issue in your life and fix it with skill and speed. Attitude is everything when it comes to developing the mindset of the problem solver, because the problem solver must believe that it can be fixed. If you don't have a sense of optimism toward the thing that you are trying to fix, then you will find the situation to be hopeless. Optimism will lead you to become resilient. You can only bounce back if you think you can win.

Think about the boxer, for a moment. When the boxer in the ring gets hit really hard and falls to the ground, he must get up in order to be able to keep fighting. But what if he is laying on the floor, believing that he is unable to win? Why would he ever stand up? Even if he is in intense pain, even if his vision is blurry and his muscles are aching, he must have, above all, optimism and a belief that he can win. Then, and only then, can he bounce back. He can hold to his resilience and stand up to fight back.

Likewise, if we don't have the optimism when looking at our problems, we will never develop the mindset of the problem solver. The problem solver's job is to look at the situation and figure out how he can solve it. But the underlying belief is that the problem *can and will* be solved. If the problem solver were to look at the situation and say "well this is hopeless," then why would they ever go about trying to fix the problem?

At the end of the day, in order to become resilient, we must develop an optimism that things will improve. We must look at the challenges in front of us as solvable and we must look at ourselves as the people who have the capability of solving it.

So how do we build a resilient mindset? How do we learn to bounce back from adversity? Here's a few things to consider:

Push yourself physically! Working out and exercising not only has great cardiovascular benefits for your body, but it also helps increase your discipline which grows your resiliency.

Don't make problems a catastrophe. When you are dealing with a problem, don't obsess over it and don't give it any power over you. By fearing the absolute worst when dealing with a problem, you are essentially letting it grow out of control. Then it starts to affect the way that you live your life. Don't let obsessive thinking drag you down!

Focus on being more flexible with your life. Oftentimes things don't work out the way we've planned and there is a strong temptation to resist what is happening. Rather than panic when you experience changes, try to look at the positives to the change. Learn to adapt to what is happening as opposed to resisting new things.

Make a point of focusing on the good things in your life, even when dealing with adversity. By developing a position of gratitude, you are inoculating yourself against stress and frustration from having to encounter hardship. Being grateful for where you are in life and having an attitude of looking on the bright side of life will ultimately decrease your stress. This will increase your natural resilience.

Embracing Challenges

One of the most crucial things that you can learn in the Art of Problem solving is learning to look at challenges as good things rather than things to be avoided. Part of our natural temperature in society today is that we have an innate desire to avoid the bad things in life. When fear rears its head, we like to retreat from the scary thing and hide somewhere safe. It's just the way our culture has raised us. Confrontation and embrace of challenge is on the lower end of the social spectrum. Passive aggressiveness and indirect confrontation, however, appear to be on the rise especially through means of communication such as email, texting and even social media.

The fact is, as a society we are starting to lose our ability to see challenge as a good and healthy thing. Why? Because challenges tend to be uncomfortable. When we experience discomfort, we immediately seek a way to escape from such feelings. This usually involves retreating from the problem at hand. Our current society is very interested in being as comfortable as possible. Convenience is usually one of the most prized possessions in the first world. The things that once were considered luxuries, such as air conditioning and computers have now worked their way into being seen as necessities. Food is readily available at every corner and the idea of skipping a meal is quickly condemned as being extremely unhealthy. The challenges that our ancestors once faced, the hardship of hunting and gathering, living in a rough and dangerous world where shelter was something you had to work hard to build, are no longer around.

Since we as people are no longer forced to live in a constant war for survival, we aren't exposed to the rigors of such challenges. When it came down to hunting, it didn't matter for our ancestors if they were overwhelmed or not. They had to hunt or they would starve to death. The threat of a predator in their midst wasn't something they could just ignore and hope it goes away. Rather they had to deal with the very real confrontation of dealing with a tribal enemy and fighting to survive. There are many benefits to modern society. We should be very thankful that modern industry and convenience allows for us to readily access food, clothing and other necessities without having to deal with the threat of death.

The problem is that there has been nothing to replace the challenges that we once faced back then. As society grows more complex, we are discovering that we have the luxury of avoiding most of our problems. Avoidance, of course, leads to disaster in the long run. Since we are able to feel good in the moment, we often choose to accept immediate gratification as opposed to feeling the discomfort of dealing with challenges.

The problem solver looks at challenges with a willingness to tackle them head on as opposed to trying to circumvent the problem. They don't let their discomfort get the best of them and they don't run away when they feel afraid or worried about a situation. They accept that they have discomfort within them but they don't stop. They embrace the challenges ahead of them as opposed to thinking of the problem as something to avoid entirely.

Our culture puts us at a natural disadvantage when it comes to dealing with discomfort because we often equate discomfort with pain. When something feels bad, we assume that it is hurting us. The reality is that our discomfort is nothing more than a signal that what we are experiencing is unpleasant. Unpleasantness isn't pain, but since we often live our lives in the search for ways to feel better, we often make the mistake of confusing the two.

Are you interested in learning to embrace obstacles in front of you, rather than shrinking away? It is not an easy process; it requires a total shift in perspective to be able to do such a thing. It's worth it, however, if you are looking to develop the mindset of a problem solver.

So how do we learn to look at obstacles as good things? Well, let's go through each step.

Change Your Perception of Discomfort

Discomfort is not a bad thing. That tenseness that you feel inside your stomach when you think of asking for that promotion, that gut-wrenching sensation you experience as you ponder asking someone out on a date, all of those feelings are natural reactions to going outside of your comfort zone. Comfort is something that you are used to. It's enjoyable and acceptable. When you are comfortable, there isn't much reason to seek change. Likewise, when you begin to experience discomfort, it is because you are in the process of some sort of change.

Discomfort isn't pain, it is merely the response to change. The problem lies in the fact that when you are experiencing change, you are often giving up something for something else. So suppose that you want to start working out. You will begin to feel a discomfort at having to wake up early each morning so that you can get your work out time. You are experiencing something new, waking up early, and it is markedly different from your old system, which was to wake up later. You might feel an immense discomfort with having to commit your time and energy to doing such a thing. However, in the long run it will actually be very good for you because you will get all of the benefits of working out.

When we begin to take action with ourselves and move outside of what is normal for us, we're going to experience some level of discomfort. If you think that these feelings of discomfort are bad, then you will shrink back and recoil in horror. You will seek a way to escape such feelings and that involves returning back to our comfort zone.

The solution to dealing with discomfort is being able to change how we look at it. Once we've started realizing that discomfort is merely an indicator that things are changing and that you are moving out of something comfortable, we can continue moving forward. If we always look at discomfort as nothing more than a bad thing, it will always hold us back.

Step Two: Realize That Obstacles Are a Part of Growth

When we encounter challenges, we are put in the precarious position of needing the skill sets to overcome them. We might not have the skills necessary to overcome the challenge or obstacle at the beginning of the problem, but if we try to focus and push ourselves to accomplish our goals, we will find ourselves growing as people.

Each time you climb over a barrier, each time you are forced to overcome an obstacle, you grow stronger for the next one. Every challenge will directly contribute to your ability to grow as a problem solver. If you allow yourself to learn from all the obstacles and challenges that are in front of you, your life will be enriched greatly. Just as discomfort is nothing more than an indicator that change is happening, so obstacles are nothing more than an opportunity for growth.

A problem solver's mindset is to look at challenges as ways for them to grow stronger. If they encounter something they can't readily solve, they grow excited at the prospect to learn something new. You can learn so much from these challenges in your life if you start to look at them as good things instead of frustrations. All it takes is a measured, focused decision to adopt a new pattern of thinking, one that looks at challenges as necessary for growth instead of something to avoid.

Run Toward Challenges

If you want to learn how to embrace challenges and become like a problem solver, then you must make the conscious effort to seek out challenges and struggles wherever you can. Building your desire to tackle a challenge head on is similar to working out a muscle. Just as you must exercise a muscle many times to make it stronger, so must you focus on seeking out challenge wherever you can in order to build the mindset of someone who is a problem solver.

What are some practical ways that you can learn to embrace challenge? Well the first step is to make the decision that you are going to seek out hardship wherever you can, so that you can build that initial reflex.

Consider the rain for a moment. What is oftentimes our reaction when it begins to rain outside? We become concerned with walking out in it, despite the fact that rain just makes us uncomfortable. Barring any serious safety issues, there's nothing that rain can do to us except make us feel a little bit wet. Someone who's looking to build up their strength and willingness to overcome challenges might see the rain as a chance to engage in a safe, accessible test of will in the face adversity. They will walk through a heavy rainstorm and endure the temporary discomfort of being cold and wet.

We will be listing out a few different ideas for how you can make a daily point of seeking out hardship and challenge in order to grow stronger. But remember, it's as much of a mindset as it is an action. You must cultivate the desire to be willing to engage in difficulty in order to be able to solve the problems better in your life.

Here are some ways that you can seek out adversity in your life:

- Take a cold shower every day for a week. In a comfort driven world, this can be an extremely effective way to learn how to push past discomfort.
- Workout in a regular manner in such a way that challenges you each time, forcing you to push past your comfort zone.
- When you have choices to choose between something that's easy and something that's hard, take the hard option.
- Take the stairs instead of the elevator. The further the stairs are, the better!
- Make a point to speak your mind when dealing with other people, don't start unnecessary fights but be willing to disagree with people in a civil manner.

Adapting the mindset of the problem solver is necessary if you're looking to be able to effectively find solutions to the things in your life that challenge you. It's not enough to simply learn how to solve a single problem, because throughout the rest of your life you're going to encounter difficulty, hardship and struggle. By adapting the mindset of the problem solver you can have an extremely sharp axe that will allow you to cut down any problem in front of you.

Chapter 7

The Science of Habits- Unraveling the Marvels of Your Brain's Habitual Symphony

Welcome to the geekiest yet most thrilling ride of our journey – Chapter 2: The Science of Habits. Get ready to don your metaphorical lab coats as we delve into the intricate dance happening inside your brain, where habits take center stage.

The Brain's Habitual Playground

Alright, let's start with the basics. Picture your brain as this bustling city, complete with its own intricate road system. Now, imagine habits as the well-worn paths, the neural highways that your brain has paved over time. These neural highways make up the habit loop, a three-step routine that is the backbone of every habit.

Cue, Routine, Reward

Routine The habitual action itself. Whether it's hitting the gym, biting: your nails, or scrolling through social media, this is the part of the loop where you're on autopilot.

Reward: Ah, the sweet taste of victory. Your brain releases a flood of feel-good chemicals, associating the completion of the routine with pleasure. This reinforces the habit loop and makes you more likely to repeat it.

Cue: This is the trigger that kickstarts the habit loop. It could be a specific time of day, an emotion, a location – anything that acts as the green light for your habit.

Meet Your Brain's Habit Heroes

Now, let's talk about the stars of the show – the basal ganglia and the prefrontal cortex. The basal ganglia is like your brain's autopilot, handling the routine part of the habit loop. It's the one that takes over when you're deep in thought or lost in a daydream.

On the other hand, the prefrontal cortex is your brain's CEO, responsible for decision-making and willpower. However, it's also a bit of a diva – it gets tired easily. Ever wondered why it's harder to resist that tempting snack in the evening? Blame it on your fatigued prefrontal cortex.

Rewiring Your Brain

Here's where things get downright magical – the concept of neuroplasticity. Your brain is like clay, constantly molding and reshaping itself based on your experiences and, you guessed it, your habits. When you repeat a habit, you're laying down new neural pathways, making it easier for your brain to travel down that familiar road in the future.

This isn't just scientific mumbo-jumbo; it's the reason you can transform a once-challenging task into second nature with enough repetition. The more you reinforce a habit, the stronger those neural connections become.

Habits and the Dopamine Dose

Now, let's talk about everyone's favorite neurotransmitter – dopamine. It's like the brain's version of confetti, released when you experience pleasure or reward. And guess what? Habits are masters at triggering dopamine release.

When you complete a routine and get that reward, your brain celebrates by showering you with dopamine. It's nature's way of saying, "Hey, great job! Let's do that again." This feel-good chemical reinforces the habit loop, making you crave that delightful sensation over and over.

A Day in the Life

To put things in perspective, let's walk through a typical day in the life of a habit loop. Imagine waking up to your alarm (cue), hitting the gym (routine), and relishing that post-workout high (reward). Before you know it, you're riding the habit loop rollercoaster without even realizing it.

But wait, there's more! Throughout the day, your brain is firing off habit loops left and right – from your morning coffee routine to your evening wind-down rituals. Your brain is a habit-forming machine, and understanding this process is the first step to harnessing its power.

Habits in Action

Now that we've uncovered the mechanics of habits, let's shine a light on the diversity of habits in our lives. There are the good ones – like exercising regularly or practicing mindfulness –

that contribute to our well-being. Then there are the not-so-great ones – the mindless snacking, the procrastination, the doom-scrolling through social media.

Understanding the habit loop helps us identify and dissect our habits, whether they're contributing positively to our lives or holding us back. It's time to be the Sherlock Holmes of our own habits, investigating the cues, routines, and rewards that make up our daily rituals.

Breaking Down the Myths

Before we wrap up this chapter, let's address a few common misconceptions about habits. Some folks believe that it takes 21 days to form a habit, while others think breaking a habit is as simple as sheer willpower. Well, folks, buckle up for a reality check.

The 21-Day Myth

Research suggests that the 21-day rule is a bit of an oversimplification. The time it takes to form a habit varies widely among individuals and depends on factors like complexity and frequency. So, don't be disheartened if your new habit doesn't stick like glue after three weeks.

The Not-So-Superhero

As for willpower, it's a finite resource. Relying solely on willpower to break a bad habit is like trying to build a skyscraper with toothpicks. Sure, it might hold up for a while, but eventually, it's going to crumble. Instead, understanding the habit loop and working with your brain's natural tendencies is a more sustainable approach.

Ready to Geek Out on Habits?

So, there you have it – the science behind the habits that shape our lives. It's like having a backstage pass to the brain's habitual symphony. Armed with this knowledge, you're not just a habit practitioner; you're a habit maestro, conducting the intricate dance of routines and rewards. As we move forward, remember: your brain is a marvel, and habits are its secret sauce. Embrace the science, fellow habit enthusiasts, and get ready to rewrite the script of your daily rituals!

Chapter 8

Forging Resilience and Growth

The journey toward mindset mastery commences with the understanding that habits are the building blocks of personal development. It goes beyond the traditional approach of setting ambitious goals and instead directs attention toward the consistent actions that lead to transformative change.

Habits are not just actions; they are the manifestation of identity. By focusing on small, incremental changes—atomic habits—one can lay the foundation for a mindset that aligns with long-term aspirations. It's about embodying the identity of the person one aspires to become and allowing habits to serve as the vehicle for that transformation.

In the pursuit of mindset mastery, the ability to navigate challenges with resilience is paramount. Mark Manson's unconventional approach in "The Subtle Art of Not Giving a F*ck" centers on embracing discomfort as a catalyst for growth. It's about adopting a stoic perspective that acknowledges the inevitability of pain and suffering while emphasizing the power of choosing one's response.

A growth-oriented mindset does not shy away from difficulties; instead, it views them as opportunities for learning and refinement. By reframing challenges as integral to the human experience, individuals can develop a mental fortitude that withstands the storms of life. The subtle art lies in choosing what truly matters and directing energy toward meaningful pursuits.

The Importance of Values: Selective Indifference

Manson's philosophy introduces the concept of selective indifference—a deliberate choice to care about what aligns with one's values and dismiss what does not. Mindset mastery involves understanding the significance of values and using them as a compass in decision-making.

By discerning between what is essential and what is trivial, individuals can cultivate a mindset that remains focused on what truly contributes to their well-being and growth. It's a practice of acknowledging that not every battle is worth fighting and that true liberation comes from aligning actions with deeply held values.

Identifying Keystone Habits: High-Impact Actions

Building Keystone Habits: Pillars of Resilience

Mindset mastery is intricately linked to the concept of keystone habits—fundamental actions that trigger a cascade of positive changes in various areas of life. These habits serve as pillars of resilience, anchoring individuals in a foundation that fosters growth.

By identifying and cultivating keystone habits, individuals can create a domino effect that extends beyond the specific actions. These habits become catalysts for broader mindset shifts, influencing how challenges are approached, decisions are made, and resilience is built. It's a strategic approach to habit formation that leverages high-impact actions for maximum transformative effect.

Sustaining Mindset Shifts

The sustainability of mindset shifts lies in the integration of rituals and consistent actions. Rituals, in this context, are intentional practices that reinforce desired behaviors and contribute to the development of a growth-oriented mindset.

Consistency is the key to habit formation, and rituals serve as the bedrock of that consistency. By incorporating rituals into daily life, individuals create a structured environment that supports the cultivation of a resilient mindset. These rituals can range from morning routines to reflective practices, each playing a crucial role in reinforcing positive habits.

Navigating the Inner Landscape

Embracing Imperfection

A resilient mindset involves radical acceptance—an acknowledgment of imperfection and a willingness to embrace the messy, unpredictable nature of life. Mindfulness, as advocated by both Clear and Manson, plays a pivotal role in this acceptance, urging individuals to be present in the moment without judgment.

By accepting the inherent flaws and uncertainties of life, individuals free themselves from the burden of unrealistic expectations. A growth-oriented mindset recognizes that failures and setbacks are not signs of inadequacy but opportunities for learning and improvement. It's about navigating the inner landscape with compassion and self-acceptance.

The Empowered Mindset

Taking ownership of one's life is a hallmark of mindset mastery. It involves a shift from a victim mentality to an empowered mindset—one that acknowledges personal agency and accountability in shaping the course of life.

The empowered mindset does not seek external validation or blame external circumstances for challenges. Instead, it recognizes the power of choice and takes deliberate actions that align with long-term goals. It's a mindset that thrives on accountability, understanding that every decision contributes to the narrative of one's life.

The Power of Self-Talk

Reflecting Mindset

Language serves as a mirror reflecting the mindset of individuals. Cultivating a growth-oriented mindset involves paying attention to the language used in self-talk and external communication.

By shifting language from a fixed to a growth orientation, individuals can reshape their perception of challenges and setbacks. It's about reframing negative self-talk, embracing a positive narrative, and consciously choosing words that reinforce a belief in personal development and resilience.

Programming the Mindset

Affirmations and visualization become powerful tools in programming a growth-oriented mindset. Affirmations are positive statements that reinforce desired beliefs and behaviors.

Visualization involves creating mental images of success and overcoming challenges.

These practices go beyond wishful thinking; they actively engage the subconscious mind in shaping beliefs and attitudes. By consistently incorporating affirmations and visualization into daily routines, individuals can reprogram their mindset to focus on possibilities, resilience, and continuous growth.

Integrating Lessons

Iterative Growth and Adaptation

Mindset mastery is an iterative process that involves mindful reflection. It's not about achieving a fixed state but about continuously adapting and growing in response to life's experiences.

Mindful reflection allows individuals to integrate lessons from successes and setbacks. It involves an honest assessment of habits, behaviors, and mindset patterns. By embracing a growth-oriented perspective in reflection, individuals can refine their approach, learn from experiences, and cultivate a mindset that evolves with each iteration.

Nurturing a Learning Mindset

Feedback becomes a valuable source of fuel for a growth-oriented mindset. It involves seeking constructive input from experiences, mentors, and the environment.

A learning mindset views feedback as an opportunity for refinement, not as a judgment of worth. By actively seeking and incorporating feedback, individuals foster a mindset that thrives on continuous improvement and adaptation. It's about approaching challenges with curiosity and a commitment to learning.

CHAPTER 9

Finding personal success and fulfilment

In our current time, a world driven by AI, internet algorithms, and cutting-edge technology. These elements have not only transformed the way we live but have also reshaped the way we communicate and think. Terms that felt unfamiliar, have integrated into our everyday vocabulary. Terms like "machine learning" and "algorithmic decision-making" are now common parlance.

Both Elon Musk and Mark Zuckerberg, play a vital role in disseminating ideas that reverberate across the digital realm. Their innovations and beliefs extend across cyberspace, touching corners of the globe. Musk's ventures in space exploration, electric vehicles, and renewable energy have sparked conversations. It went beyond reaching scientists and engineers, to everyday individuals who dream of a more sustainable future. Meanwhile, Zuckerberg's creation, Facebook (now Meta), has evolved into a global platform. It connects billions, shaping the way we interact, share information, and even engage in social activism.

Apart from these influential figures, we must recognize the significant influence held by marketing agencies. They shape our desires, creating stories that dictate what we should desire, believe, and strive for. They use psychological strategies to shape our

consumer choices and alter our perceptions of reality. So, we find ourselves influenced by the advertisements and branding efforts that saturate our digital encounters.

In this driven era, it is essential to recognize the profound impact of AI, algorithms, and technology on the way we perceive and navigate the world. Additionally, we should maintain a keen awareness of the concepts promoted by influential individuals. We need to question their implications and potential consequences. Indeed, it's vital to assess the impact of marketing agencies on moulding our wants

and convictions. We should aim to keep a sense of control in an interconnected world that's shaped by algorithms. To thrive in this changing world, we need to stay aware and actively shape the stories that define our lives.

Algorithms affect every part of our lives. These quiet makers of our online interactions guide us behind the scenes. They've shaped what we like, influenced what we watch or read. We made our digital experiences the way we like them, which is pretty amazing and sometimes makes us feel a bit uneasy.

With all the technology around us, I've been thinking: could there be algorithms that are not on our screens but are a part of our whole lives? Algorithms that don't affect

what we click on and look at, but also who we are, our families, what we achieve, and even what we don't? It's like a complicated puzzle that makes up everything about us.

Imagine trying to be successful on YouTube or having a cool Instagram account. These online places are perfect for using algorithms to do well. Smart choices about what to show and how to get people interested can help creators become famous. But there's something deeper going on: the algorithms that control these websites

are like the ones that shape our entire lives.

This leads us to a contemplative inquiry. Can the principles that drive success in the digital domain also be applied to the broader canvas of our existence? Can there be algorithms for each segment of our life? Personal growth, family dynamics, resilience in the face of adversity, and the attainment of true fulfilment? It's a question that ignites curiosity and challenges us to think beyond the confines of binary code.

As we continue our journey, let's think about the idea that our lives, like the algorithms running the internet. We may need to look at them from an algorithmic perspective to better understand, and improve. Let's see how these invisible life patterns, influenced by what we do. What we mean to do, and how everything in our lives connect, create the unique stories of each of us.

As we embark on this journey through the realm of life-altering algorithms, we must tread. In the chapters that follow, we will dive deeper into each facet of this intricate tapestry. We will explore the practical applications, ethical dilemmas, and transformative potential of these algorithms. Together, we will better understand how they shape and guide us in the pursuit of a more meaningful, values-driven, and balanced existence.

A Glimpse into the Algorithms of Life

To understand the algorithms that shape our lives, we embark on a journey through the life stories of individuals who not only understood these algorithms but also leveraged them to achieve remarkable success. Each of these stories embodies a distinct algorithm, a collection of principles and actions that propelled these individuals towards greatness.

Deciphering the Secret Rules of Success

Through these captivating life stories, our goal is to unearth the core principles that drove their success. Much like algorithms govern personalised online experiences, we'll investigate the concept that these very principles could influence the trajectory of our lives.

As we immerse ourselves in these real-life examples, we set out on a quest to extract these principles. We will transform them into algorithms that can steer us towards our own objectives and dreams. This expedition will guide us to unveil the similarities between online algorithms and the algorithms that shape our life.

Together, we will seek to comprehend the keys to achievement and fulfilment in our own unique journeys. We'll find inspiration in those who've effectively employed the principles of success to create a lasting impact on the world.

Chapter 10

Emotional Intelligence

Managing Emotions

Emotions are the vibrant hues that color the canvas of life. Understanding and managing your emotions is a powerful skill that equips you to navigate the highs and lows with resilience and grace.

Practice Mindfulness

Mindfulness is the art of being present in the moment. Engage in mindfulness practices, such as deep breathing, meditation, or simply paying attention to your surroundings. Mindfulness fosters a calm and centered emotional state.

Mindful Breathing Exercises

Incorporate short mindful breathing exercises into your daily routine. Focus on your breath, inhaling and exhaling slowly. This practice grounds you in the present moment.

Develop Emotional Resilience

Life is a roller coaster of emotions, and building emotional resilience is your seatbelt for the ride. Embrace challenges as opportunities for growth, learn from setbacks, and develop a mindset that bounces back from adversity.

Growth Mindset Reflection

Cultivate a growth mindset by viewing challenges as opportunities for learning and growth. Reflect on past challenges and identify the lessons learned and strengths gained.

Recognize Your Emotions

Emotional intelligence begins with self-awareness. Take the time to recognize and identify your emotions. Whether it's joy, anger, sadness, or excitement, understanding what you feel is the first step toward managing your emotional landscape.

Emotional Check-Ins

Conduct regular emotional check-ins with yourself. Ask, "How am I feeling right now?" This habit cultivates a heightened sense of self-awareness.

Understand the Triggers

Every emotion has its triggers. It could be a specific event, a thought, or even a particular person. Identify the triggers that evoke different emotions within you. This awareness empowers you to navigate your emotional responses more effectively.

Express Emotions Appropriately

Emotions are a natural part of the human experience, and expressing them is healthy. Learn to communicate your emotions appropriately. Whether it's sharing your joy with others or calmly expressing your frustrations, effective expression fosters understanding.

Emotion Journal

Maintain an emotion journal where you record your feelings and the ways you express them. Reflect on the outcomes of different approaches to emotional expression.

Seek Support When Needed

Managing emotions doesn't mean facing them alone. It's okay to seek support from friends, family, or professionals when emotions become overwhelming. Opening up and sharing your feelings is a sign of strength, not weakness.

Trusted Support System

Identify a trusted support system—a friend, family member, or mentor you can turn to when you need emotional support. Having someone to talk to can be immensely comforting.

Develop Coping Mechanisms

Healthy coping mechanisms are essential for managing stress and challenging emotions. Identify activities or practices that help you relax and recharge, whether it's exercising, listening to music, or spending time in nature.

Create a Relaxation Routine

Establish a relaxation routine that incorporates activities you enjoy. Whether it's reading, taking a warm bath, or practicing a hobby, a consistent routine contributes to emotional well-being.

Empathy Matters

Empathy is the bridge that connects hearts, allowing you to understand and share the feelings of others. Cultivating empathy is a cornerstone of emotional intelligence, fostering deeper and more meaningful connections with those around you.

Put Yourself in Others' Shoes

Empathy begins with the ability to imagine and understand the experiences of others. Practice putting yourself in someone else's shoes, considering their perspective, feelings, and challenges.

Empathy Exercises

Engage in empathy exercises, such as reading books from diverse perspectives, volunteering, or participating in role-playing scenarios. These activities enhance your empathetic abilities.

Listen Actively

Listening is a powerful tool for empathetic communication. When others share their experiences or feelings, practice active listening—focus on their words, ask clarifying questions, and show genuine interest in understanding their perspective.

Reflective Listening

In conversations, practice reflective listening by summarizing what the other person has shared. This not only demonstrates empathy but also ensures mutual understanding.

Practice Random Acts of Kindness

Kindness is a powerful expression of empathy. Engage in random acts of kindness, whether it's offering a helping hand, expressing gratitude, or simply being present for someone in need.

Empathy Challenge

Challenge yourself to perform one random act of kindness each day. This could be as simple as holding the door for someone or offering a genuine compliment. These small acts create ripples of empathy.

Understand Cultural Differences

Empathy extends to recognizing and respecting cultural differences. Cultivate an awareness of diverse cultural norms, practices, and perspectives. This understanding enhances your ability to connect with people from various backgrounds.

Cultural Sensitivity Training

Participate in cultural sensitivity training or workshops to deepen your understanding of different cultures. This knowledge promotes inclusive and empathetic interactions.

Validate Others' Feelings

Validation is the affirmation that someone's feelings are acknowledged and understood. When expressing empathy, validate the emotions of others. Acknowledge their experiences without judgment.

Validation Statements

Practice using validation statements such as "I can see why you would feel that way" or "Your feelings are valid." This simple act fosters a supportive and empathetic environment.

Be Present in Others' Triumphs and Challenges

True empathy extends beyond understanding during difficult times—it includes sharing in the joy of others' successes. Celebrate their achievements and be genuinely present in both their triumphs and challenges.

Thoughtful Gestures

Express empathy through thoughtful gestures. Whether it's a congratulatory note or a comforting gesture during tough times, small actions speak volumes.

Offer Support Without Judgment

Empathy is unconditional. When providing support to others, do so without judgment. Create a safe space where individuals feel free to express themselves without fear of criticism.

Practical Tip: Non-Judgmental Language

Be mindful of your language, choosing words that convey support and understanding rather than judgment. This practice fosters an environment of trust and empathy.

Resilience and Bouncing Back

Life is a series of ebbs and flows, and resilience is the life jacket that keeps you afloat during challenging times. Building resilience is a crucial aspect of emotional intelligence, allowing you to navigate setbacks and emerge stronger.

Embrace Change as an Opportunity

Change is inevitable, and resilience lies in your ability to adapt. Instead of resisting change, embrace it as an opportunity for growth and learning. See challenges as stepping stones toward a more resilient version of yourself.

Change Mindset Exercise

Challenge yourself to reframe your perspective on change. When faced with a significant change, list potential opportunities and positive outcomes it may bring. This exercise shifts your mindset toward resilience.

Develop a Positive Outlook

A positive outlook is a powerful tool in building resilience. Cultivate optimism by focusing on the silver linings in challenging situations. A positive mindset not only enhances your well-being but also fuels your resilience.

Gratitude Journal

Maintain a gratitude journal where you regularly write down things you're thankful for. This practice shifts your focus toward the positive aspects of life, fostering a more optimistic outlook.

Learn from Setbacks

Resilience is not about avoiding challenges but about learning from them. When setbacks occur, reflect on the lessons they offer. Each setback is an opportunity for growth and self-discovery.

Setback Reflection

After facing a setback, take time to reflect on what went wrong and what you can learn from the experience. This reflective practice enhances your resilience and problem-solving skills.

Develop Coping Strategies

Resilience involves having effective coping strategies to navigate stress and adversity. Identify healthy coping mechanisms that work for you, whether it's physical exercise, mindfulness, or seeking support from friends and family.

Practical Tip: Stress-Relief Toolbox

Create a stress-relief toolbox with a variety of coping mechanisms. This could include exercise routines, meditation practices, or activities that bring you joy. Having multiple tools ensures you're well-equipped to face challenges.

Cultivate a Supportive Network

A strong support network is a cornerstone of resilience. Surround yourself with friends, family, and mentors who provide emotional support during difficult times. Knowing you're not alone enhances your ability to bounce back.

Support System Evaluation

Evaluate your current support system. Identify individuals who consistently offer support and encouragement. Strengthening these connections builds a reliable foundation for resilience.

Develop Problem-Solving Skills

Resilience involves the ability to navigate challenges effectively. Develop problem-solving skills by approaching problems with a systematic mindset. Break challenges into smaller, manageable tasks and tackle them step by step.

Problem-Solving Workshops

Participate in problem-solving workshops or activities. These experiences enhance your analytical and strategic thinking, contributing to your ability to overcome obstacles.

Maintain a Healthy Lifestyle

Physical and mental well-being are interconnected. Prioritize a healthy lifestyle by getting regular exercise, maintaining a balanced diet, and ensuring sufficient sleep. A healthy body supports a resilient mind.

Wellness Check-Ins

Conduct regular wellness check-ins to assess your physical and mental well-being. Adjust your lifestyle as needed to ensure you're prioritizing your health.

Foster a Growth Mindset

A growth mindset is the belief that your abilities and intelligence can be developed through dedication and hard work. Cultivate a growth mindset, seeing challenges as opportunities to learn and improve.

Growth Mindset Affirmations

Incorporate growth mindset affirmations into your daily routine. Remind yourself that challenges are stepping stones to growth, and your efforts contribute to your ongoing development.

Set Realistic Goals

Resilience is often built through the pursuit of meaningful goals. Set realistic and achievable goals that align with your values. The sense of accomplishment from reaching these goals enhances your resilience.

SMART Goal Setting

Use the SMART criteria (Specific, Measurable, Achievable, Relevant, Time-Bound) when setting goals. This framework ensures your goals are clear, attainable, and conducive to building resilience.

Foster Adaptability

Adaptability is a key component of resilience. Develop the ability to adjust to changing circumstances and find solutions in dynamic environments. Embracing adaptability positions you to navigate life's twists and turns.

Adaptability Exercises

Engage in activities that challenge your adaptability, such as trying a new hobby, taking on a different role, or navigating unfamiliar environments. These experiences enhance your flexibility in the face of change.

Celebrate Small Wins

Resilience is built one small victory at a time. Celebrate your achievements, no matter how minor. Recognizing and acknowledging your progress fuels your motivation and resilience.

Victory Journal

Maintain a victory journal where you record your accomplishments, no matter how small. This practice provides a tangible record of your resilience and growth over time.

Closing this chapter on emotional intelligence, remember that your ability to understand, manage, and empathize with emotions is a powerful asset in navigating the complexities of life. As you continue to develop your emotional intelligence, you're not just building a skill set; you're cultivating a foundation for meaningful relationships, personal growth, and resilience.

Chapter 11

Clearly Defined Financial Objectives

The Key to Setting Financial Goals

The capacity to clearly define and communicate goals is fundamental to any successful financial journey. These objectives function as the compass points that steer all financial choices and actions. They offer a path forwards, a feeling of direction, and a system for tracking development. Setting financial goals is an introspective process that calls for a thorough understanding of one's values, desires, and ideal lifestyle. It's not just a useful exercise.

Setting Both Short-Term and Long-Term Objectives

Financial objectives differ in breadth and time span; there is no one-size-fits-all approach. Short-term objectives, which often last a year or less, can be saving for a particular item, paying off high-interest debt, or creating an emergency fund. On the other side, long-term objectives span beyond a five-year timeframe and might include significant events like becoming a homeowner, retiring, or paying for a child's school. Differentiating between short- and long-term goals is essential because it influences the tactics and tools used to accomplish them.

The Mindset Behind Goal-Setting

Setting financial objectives involves more than just the numbers; it also involves understanding the complexities of human psychology. Gaining an understanding of the psychological foundations of goal setting enables people to overcome hurdles, maintain motivation, and persevere in the face of difficulty.

Visualisation Tools and Vision Boards

It's a really effective practise to visualise reaching financial objectives. People can make concrete representations of their goals by using tools such as vision boards. These visual aids act as continuous reminders, strengthening the emotional bond with the objectives and encouraging a sense of responsibility.

A Success Road Map

Setting goals that are Specific, Measurable, Achievable, Relevant, and Time-bound (SMART) becomes essential. Financial goals become clearer and a progress roadmap is provided when they are broken down into quantifiable, specific components. Setting and achieving realistic objectives that are in line with one's values and talents gives one a feeling of direction and purpose.

Creating Your Own Financial Story: Felix's Account

To shed light on the fundamentals of goal-setting, let's go back to Felix's journey. Felix, who experienced early-life financial hardship, developed a vision of financial emancipation. His long-term vision included entrepreneurship and creating money for future generations; his short-term goals were careful budgeting and debt reduction. Felix is a wonderful example of the transformational impact of well-defined and intentional goal planning due to his steadfast adherence to the SMART criteria and his constant focus on the larger story of financial independence.

Techniques for Reaching Objectives

Setting goals is an active process that goes beyond simple expression. It demands strategic preparation, ongoing assessment, and flexibility in response to shifting conditions. In this section, we look at doable tactics for making financial objectives a reality.

Creating a Foundational Budget

A well-constructed budget is the cornerstone of achieving objectives. It gives a thorough summary of earnings, outlays, and savings as well as insights into areas that can be adjusted to better meet the set objectives. Budgeting is a freeing instrument that enables people to allocate resources consciously, not a restrictive one.

Gradual Improvement and Marking Significant Occasions

Incremental growth is a common characteristic of achieving financial goals. Larger objectives can be broken down into more manageable steps that can be celebrated. This also helps to make the process more efficient. It is essential to acknowledge and celebrate these accomplishments in order to keep motivation high and to reinforce the healthy behaviours that lead to financial success.

Financial environments are dynamic and susceptible to changes in the economy, individual situations, and unanticipated difficulties. Therefore, it is critical to have the capacity to regularly assess and modify financial objectives. When people adopt a flexible strategy and remain dedicated to the overall goal, they can successfully negotiate shifting conditions without compromising their financial goals.

Establishing specific financial goals is a fundamental first step in the greater story of financial achievement rather than an isolated action. It's a path that demands reflection, deliberate planning, and a dedication to ongoing development. Let the ideas discussed in this chapter act as a compass for you as we wrap up our investigation, pointing you in the direction of a time when your financial objectives will be more than just dreams—they will be real, measurable steps towards long-term success.

Chapter 12

Kick Your Success Addiction

This is a compelling concept urging individuals to reassess and redefine their relationship with success. Rather than perpetuating a relentless pursuit of external validation and achievements, this approach encourages a shift towards a more balanced and sustainable definition of success.

At its core, the idea challenges the societal narrative that measures success solely by traditional benchmarks such as wealth, status, or accolades. Instead, it prompts individuals to reflect on their intrinsic values, well-being, and overall life satisfaction. By doing so, one can break free from the addictive cycle of constantly chasing external validations.

This paradigm shift involves acknowledging that success is a multifaceted concept, encompassing personal growth, meaningful relationships, and a sense of purpose. It's about finding fulfillment in the journey itself rather than fixating solely on the destination.

"Kick Your Success Addiction" is an invitation to celebrate small victories, appreciate personal growth, and prioritize well-being. It encourages individuals to set realistic goals aligned with their values, fostering a healthier and more sustainable approach to personal and professional accomplishments.

In essence, the concept advocates for a mindful and intentional pursuit of success, where individuals define their own metrics and resist the societal pressure to conform to external standards. By kicking the success addiction, one can cultivate a more resilient, balanced, and genuinely fulfilling life journey.

Examining the societal pressure for continuous success

Societal pressure for continuous success is a pervasive influence that often shapes individuals' perceptions, aspirations, and behaviors. In contemporary society, there exists an implicit expectation for constant achievement and upward mobility, fostering what can be described as a "success treadmill."

This pressure is fueled by various factors, including cultural norms, media portrayals, and economic structures. The prevailing narrative often emphasizes external markers of success, such as career advancements, material wealth, and social status. As a result, individuals may feel compelled to pursue an unending cycle of achievements to meet societal expectations and gain validation.

The rise of social media further amplifies this pressure, creating a platform where curated successes are prominently displayed. The continuous stream of achievements showcased online can contribute to a sense of comparison and a fear of falling short. This can lead individuals to internalize the idea that success is a non-stop race, leaving little room for rest or self-reflection.

The pressure for continuous success can also impact mental health, contributing to stress, anxiety, and burnout. The fear of not measuring up to societal standards can lead individuals to push themselves beyond reasonable limits, neglecting their well-being in the pursuit of an ever-elusive goal.

Moreover, the societal emphasis on perpetual success can overshadow the value of failure and learning experiences. The fear of falling short may discourage risk-taking and innovation, hindering personal and collective growth.

Addressing this societal pressure requires a cultural shift towards a more holistic definition of success—one that encompasses well-being, personal fulfillment, and meaningful connections. Encouraging open conversations about the realities of success, embracing individual journeys, and celebrating diverse forms of achievement can contribute to a healthier, more balanced societal outlook. Ultimately, recognizing the multifaceted nature of success can help alleviate the undue pressure for continuous success and foster a more supportive and compassionate societal ethos.

Redefine success on one's terms and find fulfillment beyond traditional measures

This is an empowering philosophy that invites individuals to break free from conventional molds and forge paths aligned with their unique aspirations and values.

This approach encourages you to question societal norms and recognize that success is not a one-size-fits-all concept. It's an invitation to explore what truly brings meaning and satisfaction on a personal level. By embracing this mindset, you can liberate yourself from the pressures of external expectations and chart a course that resonates authentically with your inner self.

The narrative champions a holistic understanding of success that goes beyond material wealth or external validations. It prompts you to consider personal growth, well-being, and the pursuit of passions as integral components of a fulfilling life. Success becomes a dynamic, evolving journey rather than a static destination.

Finding fulfillment beyond traditional measures involves acknowledging that happiness is a deeply personal and subjective experience. You are encouraged to discover your unique sources of joy and purpose, recognizing that societal benchmarks may not necessarily align with individual desires.

The philosophy also emphasizes the importance of resilience in the face of challenges. Redefining success entails embracing setbacks not as failures but as opportunities for growth and learning. It's a call to view the entirety of one's journey — with its triumphs and obstacles — as essential to personal development.

Ultimately, this narrative serves as an empowering guide, urging you to reclaim the narrative of your lives. It's a declaration that success is most meaningful when it reflects individual values and passions. By redefining success on your terms, you embark on a journey toward a more authentic, fulfilling, and personally meaningful existence.

Chapter 13

The Discovery Process of Problem Solving

Critical Thinking:

Critical thinking is the ability to gather data and make a decision based purely off of that data. It involves research, study, verification and ultimately application of the data gathered.

In terms of problem solving, critical thinking allows for you to gather information relevant to your problem and interpret the value of it. One example of critical thinking is actually rather automatic. Going back to the example of the flat tire problem: if you had a flat tire your brain would automatically begin to retrieve any relevant data relating to a flat tire. It would begin to interpret experiences and inform you of what you know about the situation.

As discussed before, if you don't have sufficient information on the situation at hand, you won't be able to solve the problem easily. Critical thinking is an extremely important skill to have in the process of problem solving.

So how do we improve our critical thinking ability? Well you can do it by:

Reflecting more on your day and thinking through the choices you have made. By focusing on becoming more aware of your thought processes, you will be able to make better decisions in the future.

Be open minded about information. Rather than holding to one viewpoint, it's far better to look at both sides of a discussion and learn how to see the truth. Each time you analyze an argument and objectively look for truth, you are building your ability to sort through information.

Stop when making a decision and really look at all of the factors involved. Many times we tend to let our automatic decision making processes make the choice for us, so instead of thinking critically we just default to options and decisions that we are used to.

Learn to question assumptions that are being proposed to you. Especially when you're in the decision making process of solving a problem, assumptions can often be present without being challenged. By learning to look for assumptions and learning to question the validity of them, you will boost your critical thinking skills for certain.

Objectivity:

When we are looking at the discovery process, we must realize that we often take our own biases into the situation. A bias is a prejudice against a person or thing that often comes from either a negative understanding or from a negative experience. Don't discount how powerful biases can be when it comes to problem solving. If you aren't careful, a bias could quickly ruin your goals to have a solution to a problem.

Let's look at an example where bias can come into play when it comes to problem solving. Suppose that someone is trying to solve their financial situations. They are trying to use the discovery process to gather data on possible solutions. In the process of their search they come across a finance book that claims to have the solution to their debt problem. This individual says "Well I know that the Johnson's bought that book and it didn't work for them, so there's no way it'll work for me." This individual allowed their bias to prevent themselves from using a resource which very well could hold the answer to their problems.

We must be willing to look at all sources of information without letting our biases creep in. We are, of course, to use discernment and caution when it comes to believing these sources of information. But we cannot discount them just because of how we feel about the source material. An argument against the person instead of the information provided is known as an Ad Hominem attack. These are logical fallacies where we disagree with something on the person instead of on the points. Ad Hominem is usually one of the primary types of biases we can experience when we are sifting through new information. Disagreeing with a fact because you don't like the political stance of the person providing the fact is allowing your biases to get the best of you.

We are all biased in some degree. It's natural for us to have the ideas that we agree with and to be suspicious of anyone different from our point of view. But when we make the conscious effort to shelve how we feel and instead focus on what we can learn, we are opening ourselves up to information and data that we wouldn't normally look for. This can give us an advantage when it comes to being able to look at every possible solution in problem solving.

Judgment:

The final element of the discovery is learning how to have good judgment. When you are in the process of sorting through facts, ideas and concepts, it's important to be able to see what is true and tell what is false. In essence, you rely on your ability to judge in just about any situation where you have to decide between more than one outcome.

What are the things that make up good judgment? Let's take a look:

Big Picture Thinking: When you have to make a decision, it is extremely beneficial to consider the long term effects of such a choice. Oftentimes we can get bogged down in the minutia of details and only see the trees instead of the whole forest. Good judgment allows for us to focus on the whole of the problem instead of just one detail.

Thinking Realistically: If something seems too good to be true, it most likely is. A person with good judgment skills often looks for the drawback in a solution, knowing that most everything is some kind of trade off.

Gut Decisions: Sometimes something might feel off. This is our natural sense of intuition. It is our brain's ability to subconsciously put together information and signal to us that something is wrong without us explicitly knowing what is wrong. Sometimes it can be extremely beneficial to trust your gut instinct and remain cautious. You shouldn't make a serious decision just off of a feeling, but you can let those feelings give you some extra level of discernment.

Skepticism: Being overly skeptical isn't good, but having a healthy dose of skepticism in your daily thinking can assist you with making the right choices. Just because someone says something is true doesn't necessarily mean it is true.

Look for Proof: A good judge is someone who looks for proof. If a man claiming that he has a revolutionary system to get out of debt has no proof, is poor himself and those who use his system are also poor, chances are the system doesn't work so great. Trust but verify is a great policy to have in place when it comes to taking in independent information on a potential problem solver.

So with these three elements discussed, it's now time to look at a step-by-step process in which the discovery process is utilized. We will be showing you a series of actions that you can take when you begin to look at how to solve your problem. You must go slowly here, if you're looking for a quick fix to solve your problem, you are still focusing on just learning how to fix a specific problem instead of learning to adapt to a problem solver mindset.

Get the Facts

Assuming that you've broken down your problem into as many pieces as it can go, it's time for you to work on gathering all of the facts that you have available at your disposal. Write down everything that you know about the situation, don't leave anything out. For example, if one of your major problems is that your dryer isn't working properly and you aren't sure what to do, you would write a list out somewhat like this:

Fact: The Dryer isn't working

Fact: It was just fixed last week

Fact: When I try to run the dryer, it begins making a strange wheezing noise

Fact: The dryer is A Whirlpool Duet

Regardless of what the problem is, if you're looking to overcome it, you must be able to write out all of the facts that are in play. This is going to help you significantly when you begin to gather data, which is the next step.

Put Together a List of Sources of Information

Once you know what the problem is, you need to compile a central database of all the possible solutions. You must be able to know where to go for such information. For example, if you were working on fixing the dryer you would have a list of different sources of assistance in learning on solutions.

- **The whirlpool manual**
- **The Whirlpool help hot-line**

- **My neighbor who's a mechanic The Internet**
- **The mechanic who worked on the dryer last week**

By putting together, a comprehensive list of things that may potentially offer solutions, you are then able to effectively go through that list and begin gathering information on how to actually solve your problem. Please note that the discovery process is still just about educating yourself as much as possible, the third phase, the action phase, is where we will actually begin to go about solving the problem. When you choose to build the good habits of getting as educated as possible about each major problem that you face, you will be setting yourself up to live life as a problem solver!

Gathering Possible Solutions

The final step in the discovery process is putting together all of the solutions that you have come across and then working on an action plan. It might be tempting to find a solution, then try it and see it if it works one solution at a time, but this can be cumbersome and will slow you down if the first three solutions that you come across don't work.

It is more effective to be able to sit down and gather up all of the solutions that you have found, evaluate each one and then determine the order in which you will work with them. This will allow you to get fully educated on the problem and will allow for your approach to be quick and adaptive. If something doesn't work out, rather than having to go all the way back to step two, you can just go down the list to the next solution that you learned.

Here's what that list might look like if we continue using the dryer example:

- **Call the repairman and ask for his services**

- **Get a new dryer**

- **Check the door switch to see if it's working properly**

- **Unplug the dryer and test the thermal fuse**

Each solution here is ordered in such a way where the easiest solution is proposed first and then each solution after that grows more complex. By using a simple, straightforward approach to gathering information, taking inventory of the solutions and then putting together an action plan, you can learn to solve problems quickly and easily.

But what if the problems are a bit more complicated than just a broken down dryer? Well, that's where the third phase comes into place: the action phase. Let's go ahead and move onto the next chapter where we will take a look at both long-term strategy and plan implementation.

www.ingramcontent.com/pod-product-compliance
Lightning Source LLC
LaVergne TN
LVHW010224070526
838199LV00062B/4720